This
Low-Carb Meal Planner
belongs to:

_____

© Copyright 2019 by PimPom Pretty Planners – All rights reserved. Cover image and images inside: freepik.com or in public domain.

2019

JANUARY
S	M	T	W	T	F	S
		1	2	3	4	5
6	7	8	9	10	11	12
13	14	15	16	17	18	19
20	21	22	23	24	25	26
27	28	29	30	31		

FEBRUARY
S	M	T	W	T	F	S
					1	2
3	4	5	6	7	8	9
10	11	12	13	14	15	16
17	18	19	20	21	22	23
24	25	26	27	28		

MARCH
S	M	T	W	T	F	S
					1	2
3	4	5	6	7	8	9
10	11	12	13	14	15	16
17	18	19	20	21	22	23
24	25	26	27	28	29	30
31						

APRIL
S	M	T	W	T	F	S
	1	2	3	4	5	6
7	8	9	10	11	12	13
14	15	16	17	18	19	20
21	22	23	24	25	26	27
28	29	30				

MAY
S	M	T	W	T	F	S
			1	2	3	4
5	6	7	8	9	10	11
12	13	14	15	16	17	18
19	20	21	22	23	24	25
26	27	28	29	30	31	

JUNE
S	M	T	W	T	F	S
						1
2	3	4	5	6	7	8
9	10	11	12	13	14	15
16	17	18	19	20	21	22
23	24	25	26	27	28	29
30						

JULY
S	M	T	W	T	F	S
	1	2	3	4	5	6
7	8	9	10	11	12	13
14	15	16	17	18	19	20
21	22	23	24	25	26	27
28	29	30	31			

AUGUST
S	M	T	W	T	F	S
				1	2	3
4	5	6	7	8	9	10
11	12	13	14	15	16	17
18	19	20	21	22	23	24
25	26	27	28	29	30	31

SEPTEMBER
S	M	T	W	T	F	S
1	2	3	4	5	6	7
8	9	10	11	12	13	14
15	16	17	18	19	20	21
22	23	24	25	26	27	28
29	30					

OCTOBER
S	M	T	W	T	F	S
		1	2	3	4	5
6	7	8	9	10	11	12
13	14	15	16	17	18	19
20	21	22	23	24	25	26
27	28	29	30	31		

NOVEMBER
S	M	T	W	T	F	S
					1	2
3	4	5	6	7	8	9
10	11	12	13	14	15	16
17	18	19	20	21	22	23
24	25	26	27	28	29	30

DECEMBER
S	M	T	W	T	F	S
1	2	3	4	5	6	7
8	9	10	11	12	13	14
15	16	17	18	19	20	21
22	23	24	25	26	27	28
29	30	31				

How to use this Low-Carb Meal Planner?

Thanks for picking up this Meal Planner!

With this low-carb food tracker notebook, you will be able to:

- Set your health / weight loss goals
- Plan your daily meals
- Track your progress

Here's how to use it.

Begin by writing down the following:

- Your WHY
- Your GOAL
- Your STATS (weight, waist size, etc)

This is your **baseline**.

Next, it's time to **plan your meals**! This Meal Planner lets you plan and track your meals for 90 days.

At the **start of every week**, you can write down:

- Breakfast ideas
- Lunch ideas
- Dinner ideas
- Snack ideas (yes, healthy snacks are allowed!)

At the start of every week, you will also find space to write down your **shopping list**. This is great if you want to plan ahead!

For **every day**, you can write down:

- How you slept last night
- What you had for breakfast, lunch, dinner and as a snack
- How much water you drank
- Your reflection on the day + what you could improve

And at the end of every week, you'll find a page to **reflect on the week**.

Finally, at the end of every 28 days, it's time to **measure your progress**. Step on that scale and measure the (reduced) size of your waist and hips.

You GOT this!

My WHY

This is why I want to track what I eat and drink:

My GOAL:

Stats at the Start:

Weight: _____

Chest: _____

Arm: _____

Waist: _____

Hips: _____

Thigh: _____

10 Things You Can Do RIGHT NOW

- Make a cup of tea
- Go for a 10-minute walk
- Drink one less cup of coffee today
- Close your eyes. Visualize how good you will feel in 90 days
- Find a recipe for a low-carb snack
- Tell a friend about your food tracking plan. Great for accountability!
- Accept where you are in this moment. Give yourself praise for your decision to improve your health.
- Find one thing of amazing beauty. Be still and feel a sense of awe.
- Throw away unhealthy food
- Find your tribe. Go online (Facebook; YouTube) and find likeminded people!

FOOD IDEAS - Week 1

Breakfast:

Lunch:

Dinner:

Snacks:

SHOPPING LIST - Week 1

Day ①

How did I sleep?

Breakfast:

Lunch:

Dinner:

Snacks:

Water:

How was my day?

What could I improve tomorrow?

Day ②

How did I sleep?

Breakfast:

Lunch:

Dinner:

Snacks:

Water:

How was my day?

What could I improve tomorrow?

Day ③

How did I sleep?   😃 🙂 😐 🙁 😣

Breakfast:

Lunch:

Dinner:

Snacks:

Water: 🥛🥛🥛🥛🥛🥛🥛🥛🥛🥛🥛🥛🥛🥛

How was my day?

What could I improve tomorrow?

Day 4

How did I sleep?

Breakfast:

Lunch:

Dinner:

Snacks:

Water:

How was my day?

What could I improve tomorrow?

Day 5

How did I sleep?　😀　🙂　😐　🙁　😣

Breakfast:　　　　　　　Lunch:

Dinner:　　　　　　　　Snacks:

Water: 🥛🥛🥛🥛🥛🥛🥛🥛🥛🥛🥛🥛🥛🥛

How was my day?

What could I improve tomorrow?

Day 6

How did I sleep?   😃 🙂 😐 🙁 😣

Breakfast: Lunch:

_____   _____
_____   _____
_____   _____
_____   _____
_____   _____

Dinner: Snacks:

_____   _____
_____   _____
_____   _____
_____   _____

Water: 🥛🥛🥛🥛🥛🥛🥛🥛🥛🥛🥛🥛

How was my day?

_____
_____
_____

What could I improve tomorrow?

_____
_____
_____

Day (7)

How did I sleep? 😄 🙂 😐 🙁 😣

Breakfast: *Lunch:*

_____   _____
_____   _____
_____   _____
_____   _____

Dinner: *Snacks:*

_____   _____
_____   _____
_____   _____
_____   _____

Water: 🥛🥛🥛🥛🥛🥛🥛🥛🥛🥛🥛🥛🥛

How was my day?

_____
_____

What could I improve tomorrow?

_____
_____

Reflection - Week 1

How was my week?

What lesson did I learn?

What change would make next week (even) better?

FOOD IDEAS - Week 2

Breakfast:

Lunch:

Dinner:

Snacks:

SHOPPING LIST – Week 2

THE
BEST WAY
to
PREDICT
the
◄ future ►
is
TO *create* IT

Day 8

How did I sleep?

Breakfast:

Lunch:

Dinner:

Snacks:

Water:

How was my day?

What could I improve tomorrow?

Day ⑨

How did I sleep?   😛 🙂 😐 🙁 😖

Breakfast: Lunch:

_____   _____
_____   _____
_____   _____
_____   _____

Dinner: Snacks:

_____   _____
_____   _____
_____   _____
_____   _____

Water: ⊔⊔⊔⊔⊔⊔⊔⊔⊔⊔⊔⊔⊔⊔

How was my day?

_____
_____
_____

What could I improve tomorrow?

_____
_____
_____

Day 10

How did I sleep? 😀 🙂 😐 🙁 😣

Breakfast:

Lunch:

Dinner:

Snacks:

Water:

How was my day?

What could I improve tomorrow?

Day (11)

How did I sleep?   😐 🙂 😐 🙁 😣

Breakfast: Lunch:

_____   _____
_____   _____
_____   _____
_____   _____
_____   _____

Dinner: Snacks:

_____   _____
_____   _____
_____   _____
_____   _____

Water: 🥛🥛🥛🥛🥛🥛🥛🥛🥛🥛🥛🥛🥛🥛

How was my day?

_____
_____
_____

What could I improve tomorrow?

_____
_____
_____

Day 12

How did I sleep?

Breakfast:

Lunch:

Dinner:

Snacks:

Water:

How was my day?

What could I improve tomorrow?

Day (13)

How did I sleep? 😀 🙂 😐 🙁 😣

Breakfast: Lunch:

_____   _____
_____   _____
_____   _____
_____   _____

Dinner: Snacks:

_____   _____
_____   _____
_____   _____
_____   _____

Water: ⊔⊔⊔⊔⊔⊔⊔⊔⊔⊔⊔⊔⊔⊔

How was my day?

_____
_____
_____

What could I improve tomorrow?

_____
_____
_____

Day (14)

How did I sleep?   😀 🙂 😐 🙁 😖

Breakfast: Lunch:

_____   _____
_____   _____
_____   _____
_____   _____

Dinner: Snacks:

_____   _____
_____   _____
_____   _____
_____   _____

Water: 🥛🥛🥛🥛🥛🥛🥛🥛🥛🥛🥛🥛

How was my day?

_____
_____
_____

What could I improve tomorrow?

_____
_____
_____

Reflection - Week 2

How was my week?

_____

_____

_____

_____

_____

What lesson did I learn?

_____

_____

_____

_____

_____

What change would make next week (even) better?

_____

_____

_____

_____

_____

FOOD IDEAS - Week 3

Breakfast:

Lunch:

Dinner:

Snacks:

SHOPPING LIST - Week 3

Day (15)

How did I sleep?   😀 🙂 😐 🙁 😣

Breakfast: Lunch:

_____   _____
_____   _____
_____   _____
_____   _____

Dinner: Snacks:

_____   _____
_____   _____
_____   _____
_____   _____

Water: ⊔⊔⊔⊔⊔⊔⊔⊔⊔⊔⊔⊔⊔⊔

How was my day?

_____
_____
_____

What could I improve tomorrow?

_____
_____
_____

Day 16

How did I sleep?

Breakfast:

Lunch:

Dinner:

Snacks:

Water:

How was my day?

What could I improve tomorrow?

Day (17)

How did I sleep?   🙂 🙂 😐 🙁 😖

Breakfast:

Lunch:

Dinner:

Snacks:

Water:

How was my day?

What could I improve tomorrow?

Day 18

How did I sleep?

Breakfast:

_____

_____

_____

_____

Lunch:

_____

_____

_____

_____

Dinner:

_____

_____

_____

_____

Snacks:

_____

_____

_____

_____

Water:

How was my day?

_____

_____

_____

What could I improve tomorrow?

_____

_____

_____

Day (19)

How did I sleep?   😀 🙂 😐 🙁 😣

Breakfast:

Lunch:

Dinner:

Snacks:

Water: 🥛🥛🥛🥛🥛🥛🥛🥛🥛🥛🥛🥛

How was my day?

What could I improve tomorrow?

Day 20

How did I sleep?

Breakfast:

Lunch:

Dinner:

Snacks:

Water:

How was my day?

What could I improve tomorrow?

Day ㉑

How did I sleep?   😀 🙂 😐 🙁 😣

Breakfast: *Lunch:*

_____   _____
_____   _____
_____   _____
_____   _____

Dinner: *Snacks:*

_____   _____
_____   _____
_____   _____
_____   _____

Water: 🥛🥛🥛🥛🥛🥛🥛🥛🥛🥛🥛🥛🥛

How was my day?

_____
_____
_____

What could I improve tomorrow?

_____
_____
_____

Reflection - Week 3

How was my week?

What lesson did I learn?

What change would make next week (even) better?

FOOD IDEAS - Week 4

Breakfast:

Lunch:

Dinner:

Snacks:

SHOPPING LIST - Week 4

Day 22

How did I sleep? 😀 🙂 😐 🙁 😣

Breakfast: **Lunch:**

Dinner: **Snacks:**

Water: 🥛🥛🥛🥛🥛🥛🥛🥛🥛🥛🥛🥛🥛🥛

How was my day?

What could I improve tomorrow?

Day 23

How did I sleep?   😀 🙂 😐 🙁 😣

Breakfast: Lunch:

_____   _____
_____   _____
_____   _____
_____   _____
_____   _____

Dinner: Snacks:

_____   _____
_____   _____
_____   _____
_____   _____

Water: ⊔⊔⊔⊔⊔⊔⊔⊔⊔⊔⊔⊔⊔⊔

How was my day?

_____
_____
_____

What could I improve tomorrow?

_____
_____
_____

Day 24

How did I sleep?

Breakfast:

Lunch:

Dinner:

Snacks:

Water:

How was my day?

What could I improve tomorrow?

Day 25

How did I sleep?

Breakfast:

Lunch:

Dinner:

Snacks:

Water:

How was my day?

What could I improve tomorrow?

Day (26)

How did I sleep?

Breakfast:

Lunch:

Dinner:

Snacks:

Water:

How was my day?

What could I improve tomorrow?

Day (27)

How did I sleep?

Breakfast:

Lunch:

Dinner:

Snacks:

Water:

How was my day?

What could I improve tomorrow?

Day (28)

How did I sleep? 😃 🙂 😐 🙁 😣

Breakfast:

Lunch:

Dinner:

Snacks:

Water: ⊔⊔⊔⊔⊔⊔⊔⊔⊔⊔⊔⊔⊔⊔

How was my day?

What could I improve tomorrow?

Reflection - Week 4

How was my week?

What lesson did I learn?

What change would make next week (even) better?

Stats After 4 Weeks:

Weight: _____

Chest: _____

Arm: _____

Waist: _____

Hips: _____

Thigh: _____

Opportunity doesn't knock,
....
➥ *build* ➥
@
DOOR

FOOD IDEAS - Week 5

Breakfast:

Lunch:

Dinner:

Snacks:

SHOPPING LIST – Week 5

Day 29

How did I sleep?

Breakfast:

Lunch:

Dinner:

Snacks:

Water:

How was my day?

What could I improve tomorrow?

Day 30

How did I sleep?   😀 🙂 😐 🙁 😣

Breakfast: Lunch:

_____   _____
_____   _____
_____   _____
_____   _____

Dinner: Snacks:

_____   _____
_____   _____
_____   _____
_____   _____

Water: 🥛🥛🥛🥛🥛🥛🥛🥛🥛🥛🥛🥛🥛🥛

How was my day?

_____
_____
_____

What could I improve tomorrow?

_____
_____
_____

Day (31)

How did I sleep? 😀 🙂 😐 🙁 😣

Breakfast:

Lunch:

Dinner:

Snacks:

Water: 🥛🥛🥛🥛🥛🥛🥛🥛🥛🥛🥛🥛🥛🥛

How was my day?

What could I improve tomorrow?

Day 32

How did I sleep?

Breakfast:

Lunch:

Dinner:

Snacks:

Water:

How was my day?

What could I improve tomorrow?

Day (33)

How did I sleep?   🙂 🙂 😐 😟 😣

Breakfast: | Lunch:

Dinner: | Snacks:

Water: 🥛🥛🥛🥛🥛🥛🥛🥛🥛🥛🥛🥛🥛

How was my day?

What could I improve tomorrow?

Day 34

How did I sleep? 😀 🙂 😐 🙁 😣

Breakfast:

_____
_____
_____
_____

Lunch:

_____
_____
_____
_____

Dinner:

_____
_____
_____
_____

Snacks:

_____
_____
_____
_____

Water: 🥛🥛🥛🥛🥛🥛🥛🥛🥛🥛🥛🥛

How was my day?

_____
_____
_____

What could I improve tomorrow?

_____
_____
_____

Day (35)

How did I sleep? 😀 🙂 😐 🙁 😣

Breakfast:

Lunch:

Dinner:

Snacks:

Water: 🥛🥛🥛🥛🥛🥛🥛🥛🥛🥛🥛🥛

How was my day?

What could I improve tomorrow?

Reflection - Week 5

How was my week?

What lesson did I learn?

What change would make next week (even) better?

FOOD IDEAS - Week 6

Breakfast:

Lunch:

Dinner:

Snacks:

SHOPPING LIST – Week 6

Day (36)

How did I sleep? 😀 🙂 😐 🙁 😣

Breakfast: | Lunch:

Dinner: | Snacks:

Water: 🥛🥛🥛🥛🥛🥛🥛🥛🥛🥛🥛🥛

How was my day?

What could I improve tomorrow?

Day 37

How did I sleep?   😃 🙂 😐 🙁 😣

Breakfast: Lunch:

_____   _____
_____   _____
_____   _____
_____   _____

Dinner: Snacks:

_____   _____
_____   _____
_____   _____
_____   _____

Water: ⎕⎕⎕⎕⎕⎕⎕⎕⎕⎕⎕⎕⎕⎕⎕⎕

How was my day?

_____
_____
_____

What could I improve tomorrow?

_____
_____
_____

Day (38)

How did I sleep?

Breakfast:

Lunch:

Dinner:

Snacks:

Water:

How was my day?

What could I improve tomorrow?

Day 39

How did I sleep?

Breakfast: Lunch:

Dinner: Snacks:

Water:

How was my day?

What could I improve tomorrow?

Day 40

How did I sleep?

Breakfast:

Lunch:

Dinner:

Snacks:

Water:

How was my day?

What could I improve tomorrow?

Day 41

How did I sleep? 😄 🙂 😐 🙁 😖

Breakfast:

Lunch:

Dinner:

Snacks:

Water: 🥛🥛🥛🥛🥛🥛🥛🥛

How was my day?

What could I improve tomorrow?

Day 42

How did I sleep?

Breakfast:

Lunch:

Dinner:

Snacks:

Water:

How was my day?

What could I improve tomorrow?

Reflection - Week 6

How was my week?

_____

_____

_____

_____

_____

What lesson did I learn?

_____

_____

_____

_____

_____

What change would make next
week (even) better?

_____

_____

_____

_____

_____

FOOD IDEAS - Week 7

Breakfast:

Lunch:

Dinner:

Snacks:

SHOPPING LIST – Week 7

Day 43

How did I sleep?

Breakfast:

Lunch:

Dinner:

Snacks:

Water:

How was my day?

What could I improve tomorrow?

Day 44

How did I sleep?

Breakfast:

Lunch:

Dinner:

Snacks:

Water:

How was my day?

What could I improve tomorrow?

Day 45

How did I sleep?

Breakfast:

Lunch:

Dinner:

Snacks:

Water:

How was my day?

What could I improve tomorrow?

Day 46

How did I sleep?   😀 🙂 😐 🙁 😣

Breakfast: Lunch:

Dinner: Snacks:

Water: 🥛🥛🥛🥛🥛🥛🥛🥛🥛🥛🥛🥛

How was my day?

What could I improve tomorrow?

Day (47)

How did I sleep?   😃 🙂 😐 🙁 😣

Breakfast:

Lunch:

Dinner:

Snacks:

Water: ⎕⎕⎕⎕⎕⎕⎕⎕⎕⎕⎕⎕⎕⎕⎕

How was my day?

What could I improve tomorrow?

Day 48

How did I sleep? 😀 🙂 😐 🙁 😣

Breakfast:

Lunch:

Dinner:

Snacks:

Water:

How was my day?

What could I improve tomorrow?

Day (49)

How did I sleep? 😀 😊 😐 ☹️ 😣

Breakfast:

Lunch:

Dinner:

Snacks:

Water: 🥛🥛🥛🥛🥛🥛🥛🥛🥛🥛🥛🥛🥛🥛

How was my day?

What could I improve tomorrow?

Reflection - Week 7

How was my week?

What lesson did I learn?

What change would make next week (even) better?

FOOD IDEAS - Week 8

Breakfast:

Lunch:

Dinner:

Snacks:

SHOPPING LIST - Week 8

Day 50

How did I sleep?　😀 🙂 😐 🙁 😣

Breakfast:　　　　　　　Lunch:

_____　　_____
_____　　_____
_____　　_____
_____　　_____

Dinner:　　　　　　　　Snacks:

_____　　_____
_____　　_____
_____　　_____
_____　　_____

Water:　🥛🥛🥛🥛🥛🥛🥛🥛🥛🥛🥛🥛🥛🥛

How was my day?

_____
_____
_____

What could I improve tomorrow?

_____
_____
_____

Day 51

How did I sleep?   😃 🙂 😐 🙁 😣

Breakfast: Lunch:

_____   _____
_____   _____
_____   _____
_____   _____
_____   _____

Dinner: Snacks:

_____   _____
_____   _____
_____   _____
_____   _____

Water: 🥛🥛🥛🥛🥛🥛🥛🥛🥛🥛🥛🥛🥛🥛

How was my day?

_____
_____
_____

What could I improve tomorrow?

_____
_____
_____

Day (52)

How did I sleep?   😃 🙂 😐 🙁 😣

Breakfast: Lunch:

_____   _____
_____   _____
_____   _____
_____   _____
_____

Dinner: Snacks:

_____   _____
_____   _____
_____   _____
_____   _____

Water: ⊔ ⊔ ⊔ ⊔ ⊔ ⊔ ⊔ ⊔ ⊔ ⊔ ⊔ ⊔ ⊔ ⊔

How was my day?

_____
_____
_____

What could I improve tomorrow?

_____
_____
_____

Day 53

How did I sleep?   😃 🙂 😐 🙁 😣

Breakfast:

_____

Lunch:

_____

Dinner:

_____

Snacks:

_____

Water: 🥛🥛🥛🥛🥛🥛🥛🥛🥛🥛🥛🥛

How was my day?

_____

What could I improve tomorrow?

_____

Day (54)

How did I sleep?   😀 🙂 😐 🙁 😣

Breakfast:

_____
_____
_____
_____
_____

Lunch:

_____
_____
_____
_____
_____

Dinner:

_____
_____
_____
_____
_____

Snacks:

_____
_____
_____
_____
_____

Water: 🥛🥛🥛🥛🥛🥛🥛🥛🥛🥛🥛🥛🥛🥛

How was my day?

_____
_____
_____

What could I improve tomorrow?

_____
_____
_____

Day 55

How did I sleep?

Breakfast:

_____
_____
_____
_____

Lunch:

_____
_____
_____
_____

Dinner:

_____
_____
_____
_____

Snacks:

_____
_____
_____
_____

Water:

How was my day?

_____
_____
_____

What could I improve tomorrow?

_____
_____
_____

Day (56)

How did I sleep?   😀 🙂 😐 🙁 😣

Breakfast: Lunch:

_____   _____
_____   _____
_____   _____
_____   _____

Dinner: Snacks:

_____   _____
_____   _____
_____   _____
_____   _____

Water: 🥛🥛🥛🥛🥛🥛🥛🥛🥛🥛🥛🥛🥛🥛

How was my day?

_____
_____
_____

What could I improve tomorrow?

_____
_____
_____

Reflection - Week 8

How was my week?

What lesson did I learn?

What change would make next week (even) better?

Stats After 8 Weeks:

Weight: _____

Chest: _____

Arm: _____

Waist: _____

Hips: _____

Thigh: _____

FOOD IDEAS - Week 9

Breakfast:

Lunch:

Dinner:

Snacks:

SHOPPING LIST - Week 9

Day 57

How did I sleep?　😃 😊 😐 🙁 😣

Breakfast:

Lunch:

Dinner:

Snacks:

Water:

How was my day?

What could I improve tomorrow?

Day 58

How did I sleep?

Breakfast:

Lunch:

Dinner:

Snacks:

Water:

How was my day?

What could I improve tomorrow?

Day 59

How did I sleep? 🙂 🙂 😐 🙁 😖

Breakfast:

_____

Lunch:

_____

Dinner:

_____

Snacks:

_____

Water: 🥛🥛🥛🥛🥛🥛🥛🥛🥛🥛🥛🥛🥛🥛🥛

How was my day?

_____

What could I improve tomorrow?

_____

Day 60

How did I sleep? 😃 🙂 😐 🙁 😣

Breakfast:

Lunch:

Dinner:

Snacks:

Water: 🥛🥛🥛🥛🥛🥛🥛🥛🥛🥛🥛🥛🥛🥛🥛

How was my day?

What could I improve tomorrow?

Day (61)

How did I sleep?   😀 🙂 😐 😟 😣

Breakfast: Lunch:

_____   _____
_____   _____
_____   _____
_____   _____
_____   _____

Dinner: Snacks:

_____   _____
_____   _____
_____   _____
_____   _____
_____   _____

Water: ⊔ ⊔ ⊔ ⊔ ⊔ ⊔ ⊔ ⊔ ⊔ ⊔ ⊔ ⊔ ⊔ ⊔

How was my day?

_____
_____
_____

What could I improve tomorrow?

_____
_____
_____

Day 62

How did I sleep?

Breakfast:

Lunch:

Dinner:

Snacks:

Water:

How was my day?

What could I improve tomorrow?

Day 63

How did I sleep?

Breakfast:

Lunch:

Dinner:

Snacks:

Water:

How was my day?

What could I improve tomorrow?

Reflection - Week 9

How was my week?

What lesson did I learn?

What change would make next week (even) better?

FOOD IDEAS - Week 10

Breakfast:

Lunch:

Dinner:

Snacks:

SHOPPING LIST - Week 10

Day (64)

How did I sleep? 😃 🙂 😐 🙁 😖

Breakfast: Lunch:

_____   _____
_____   _____
_____   _____
_____   _____
_____   _____

Dinner: Snacks:

_____   _____
_____   _____
_____   _____
_____   _____

Water: ⊔⊔⊔⊔⊔⊔⊔⊔⊔⊔⊔⊔⊔⊔

How was my day?

_____
_____
_____

What could I improve tomorrow?

_____
_____
_____

Day 65

How did I sleep?   😀 😊 😐 🙁 😣

Breakfast:

Lunch:

Dinner:

Snacks:

Water: 🥛🥛🥛🥛🥛🥛🥛🥛🥛🥛🥛🥛🥛🥛

How was my day?

What could I improve tomorrow?

Day 66

How did I sleep?

😃 🙂 😐 🙁 😣

Breakfast:

Lunch:

Dinner:

Snacks:

Water:

How was my day?

What could I improve tomorrow?

Day 67

How did I sleep?   😃 🙂 😐 🙁 😣

Breakfast:

Lunch:

Dinner:

Snacks:

Water: 🥛🥛🥛🥛🥛🥛🥛🥛🥛🥛🥛🥛🥛🥛

How was my day?

What could I improve tomorrow?

Day (68)

How did I sleep?

Breakfast:

Lunch:

Dinner:

Snacks:

Water:

How was my day?

What could I improve tomorrow?

Day 69

How did I sleep?

Breakfast:

Lunch:

Dinner:

Snacks:

Water:

How was my day?

What could I improve tomorrow?

Day 70

How did I sleep? 😃 🙂 😐 🙁 😖

Breakfast:

Lunch:

Dinner:

Snacks:

Water: 🥛🥛🥛🥛🥛🥛🥛🥛🥛🥛🥛🥛

How was my day?

What could I improve tomorrow?

Reflection - Week 10

How was my week?

What lesson did I learn?

What change would make next
week (even) better?

FOOD IDEAS - Week 11

Breakfast:

Lunch:

Dinner:

Snacks:

SHOPPING LIST – Week 11

Day (71)

How did I sleep? 😄 🙂 😐 🙁 😣

Breakfast:

Lunch:

Dinner:

Snacks:

Water: 🥛🥛🥛🥛🥛🥛🥛🥛🥛🥛🥛🥛🥛🥛

How was my day?

What could I improve tomorrow?

Day 72

How did I sleep?

Breakfast:

Lunch:

Dinner:

Snacks:

Water:

How was my day?

What could I improve tomorrow?

Day 73

How did I sleep?   😀 🙂 😐 🙁 😣

Breakfast:

Lunch:

Dinner:

Snacks:

Water:

How was my day?

What could I improve tomorrow?

Day (74)

How did I sleep?   😄 🙂 😐 😠 😣

Breakfast: Lunch:

_____   _____
_____   _____
_____   _____
_____   _____
_____   _____

Dinner: Snacks:

_____   _____
_____   _____
_____   _____
_____   _____

Water: ⊔⊔⊔⊔⊔⊔⊔⊔⊔⊔⊔⊔⊔⊔

How was my day?

_____
_____
_____

What could I improve tomorrow?

_____
_____
_____

Day 75

How did I sleep?

Breakfast:

_____

Lunch:

_____

Dinner:

_____

Snacks:

_____

Water:

How was my day?

_____

What could I improve tomorrow?

_____

Day 76

How did I sleep?

Breakfast:

_____
_____
_____
_____

Lunch:

_____
_____
_____
_____

Dinner:

_____
_____
_____
_____

Snacks:

_____
_____
_____
_____

Water:

How was my day?

_____
_____
_____

What could I improve tomorrow?

_____
_____
_____

Day 77

How did I sleep?

Breakfast:

Lunch:

Dinner:

Snacks:

Water:

How was my day?

What could I improve tomorrow?

Reflection - Week 11

How was my week?

What lesson did I learn?

What change would make next week (even) better?

FOOD IDEAS - Week 12

Breakfast:

Lunch:

Dinner:

Snacks:

SHOPPING LIST – Week 12

Day 78

How did I sleep? 😃 🙂 😐 🙁 😣

Breakfast:

Lunch:

Dinner:

Snacks:

Water: 🥛🥛🥛🥛🥛🥛🥛🥛🥛🥛🥛🥛🥛

How was my day?

What could I improve tomorrow?

Day 79

How did I sleep?

Breakfast:

Lunch:

Dinner:

Snacks:

Water:

How was my day?

What could I improve tomorrow?

Day (80)

How did I sleep? 😀 🙂 😐 🙁 😖

Breakfast:

_____

Lunch:

_____

Dinner:

_____

Snacks:

_____

Water: 🥛🥛🥛🥛🥛🥛🥛🥛🥛🥛🥛🥛🥛🥛

How was my day?

_____

What could I improve tomorrow?

_____

Day 81

How did I sleep?

Breakfast:

Lunch:

Dinner:

Snacks:

Water:

How was my day?

What could I improve tomorrow?

Day (82)

How did I sleep?

Breakfast:

Lunch:

Dinner:

Snacks:

Water:

How was my day?

What could I improve tomorrow?

Day 83

How did I sleep?

Breakfast:

Lunch:

Dinner:

Snacks:

Water:

How was my day?

What could I improve tomorrow?

Day 84

How did I sleep?

Breakfast:

Lunch:

Dinner:

Snacks:

Water:

How was my day?

What could I improve tomorrow?

Reflection - Week 12

How was my week?

What lesson did I learn?

What change would make next week (even) better?

Stats After 12 Weeks:

Weight: _____

Chest: _____

Arm: _____

Waist: _____

Hips: _____

Thigh: _____

Want to keep going?

You are (almost) at the end of this meal planner.

Well done!

But...you're about to run out of space. And you may want to continue with your meal tracking habit.

Don't worry!

On the next pages, you will find a **BONUS** week. This gives you time to get your hands on a new planner.

Curious about our other planners? Then check out our author page on Amazon.

Let's continue.

FOOD IDEAS - Week 13

Breakfast:

Lunch:

Dinner:

Snacks:

SHOPPING LIST – Week 13

Day 85

How did I sleep?

Breakfast:

Lunch:

Dinner:

Snacks:

Water:

How was my day?

What could I improve tomorrow?

Day 86

How did I sleep? 😀 🙂 😐 🙁 😣

Breakfast:

Lunch:

Dinner:

Snacks:

Water:

How was my day?

What could I improve tomorrow?

Day 87

How did I sleep?

Breakfast:

Lunch:

Dinner:

Snacks:

Water:

How was my day?

What could I improve tomorrow?

Day (88)

How did I sleep?   😃 🙂 😐 🙁 😣

Breakfast: Lunch:

_____   _____
_____   _____
_____   _____
_____   _____
_____

Dinner: Snacks:

_____   _____
_____   _____
_____   _____
_____   _____
_____

Water: 🥛🥛🥛🥛🥛🥛🥛🥛🥛🥛🥛🥛🥛🥛

How was my day?

_____
_____
_____

What could I improve tomorrow?

_____
_____
_____

Day (89)

How did I sleep?   😀 🙂 😐 🙁 😖

Breakfast: Lunch:

_____   _____
_____   _____
_____   _____
_____   _____
_____   _____

Dinner: Snacks:

_____   _____
_____   _____
_____   _____
_____   _____
_____   _____

Water: 🥛🥛🥛🥛🥛🥛🥛🥛🥛🥛🥛🥛🥛🥛🥛🥛

How was my day?

_____
_____
_____

What could I improve tomorrow?

_____
_____
_____

Day 90

How did I sleep?

Breakfast:

Lunch:

Dinner:

Snacks:

Water:

How was my day?

What could I improve tomorrow?

Day 91

How did I sleep?

Breakfast:

Lunch:

Dinner:

Snacks:

Water:

How was my day?

What could I improve tomorrow?

Reflection - Week 13

How was my week?

What lesson did I learn?

What change would make next week (even) better?

BOOM: You Did It!

Congratulations: You tracked your meals for a whopping **3 months**!

You are AWESOME!

Did you achieve the goal you set for yourself? You must have had a **strong WHY** to stay on course.

Is this where it ends?

No. This is only the beginning. The beginning of a new **YOU**. It's much harder to get started than to keep going.

You have now developed this amazing habit of eating healthy and keeping your weight in check. You can do anything you set your mind to.

So, what's next for you?

Don't wait for the

Perfect Moment

Take the moment
······ AND ······

Make It

Perfect

Did you like this Low-Carb Meal Planner?

If you enjoyed this meal planner, I would like to ask you for a favor.

Could you please leave a review on Amazon?

Reviews are the lifeblood of independent authors. I know, you're short on time. But I would really appreciate even just a few sentences!

The more reviews this meal planner gets, the more people will be able to find it and improve their health by tracking what they eat.

Thank you again for using this meal planner. Good luck with staying fit and healthy!

I'm rooting for you...

Made in the USA
Middletown, DE
28 July 2019